I Love Someone with Type 1 Diabetes

A BOOK ABOUT A YOUNG GIRL WITH TYPE 1 DIABETES

BY SOPHIA XENAKIS

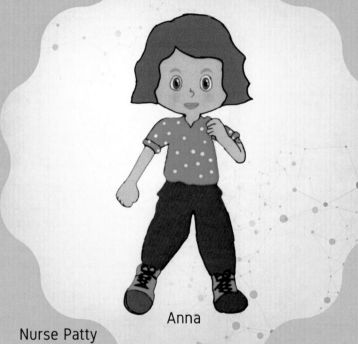

Anna

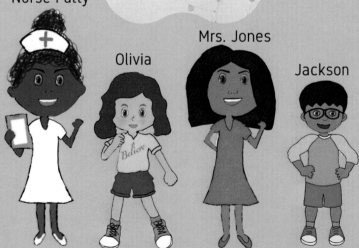

Nurse Patty

Olivia

Mrs. Jones

Jackson

To Grammy for all of your love and support.

Text copyright © 2023 by Sophia Xenakis
Illustrations copyright © 2023 by Sophia Xenakis

ISBN 979-8-9880001-0-5 (paperback)
ISBN 979-8-9880001-1-2 (e-book)
Library of Congress Control Number: 2023904773

10 9 8 7 6 5 4 3 2 1
10 9 8 7 6 5 4 3 2 1

Sophia Xenakis
New Providence, NJ

Hi, my name is Olivia, and my younger sister Anna has type 1 diabetes. Before you ask, no she didn't get diabetes from eating too much sugar. The cause of type 1 diabetes is unknown. Type 1 diabetes cannot be prevented and you cannot share it with others so don't be shy about giving lots of hugs!

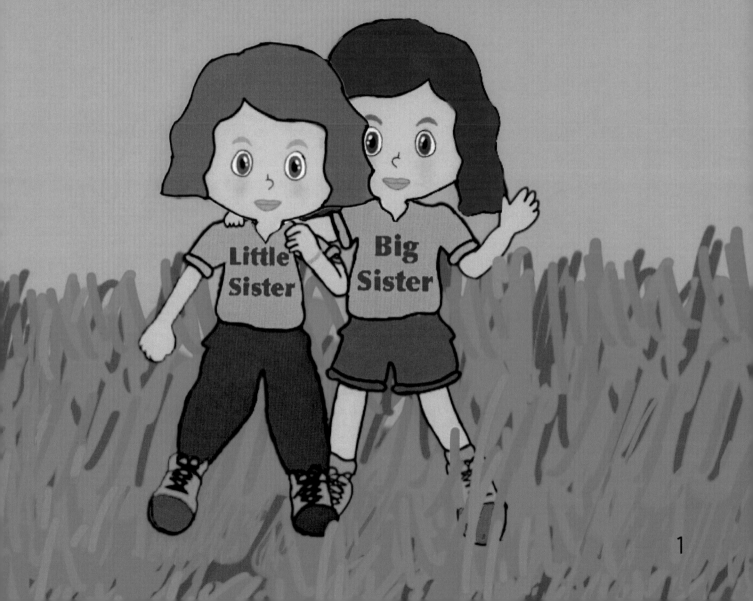

Anna's doctor thought she might have type 1 diabetes when she went to visit him. She was always hungry and thirsty and was losing weight. Anna was also always tired and peeing all of the time. These are common symptoms of people with type 1 diabetes so her doctor decided to test Anna's blood for this disease.

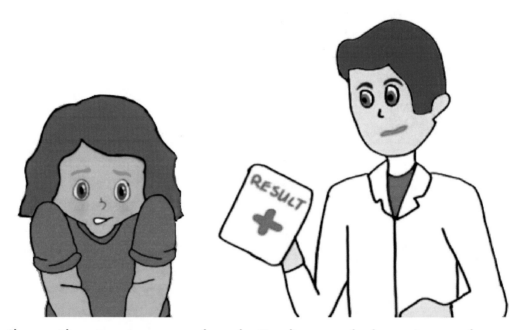

When the test came back it showed that Anna has type 1 diabetes. She was so scared. But now that she has learned about type 1 diabetes she is no longer afraid.

I am so proud of Anna.
I do everything I can to
help her. Anna feels safe
when people understand
about type 1 diabetes.
I would like to teach you
about type 1 diabetes, so
when you meet someone
with type 1 diabetes you
can help them feel safe.

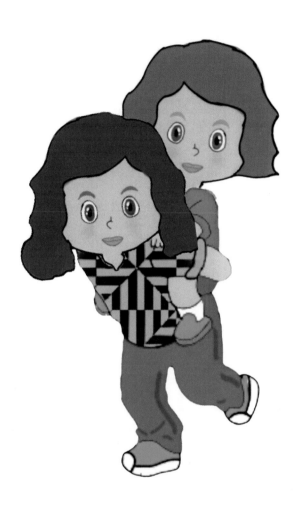

Type 1 diabetes means the pancreas does not produce insulin for the body to maintain the proper sugar level it needs. Controlling blood sugar is important because it keeps other organs like your brain and kidneys working properly.

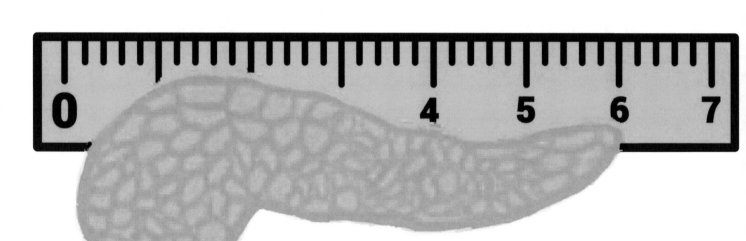

4

Challenge Box

The kidneys are in the middle of the abdomen towards your back. In this picture they are partially covered by other organs. The kidneys are the same shape as a popular candy. Can you guess what candy?
HINT: The candy looks like this.

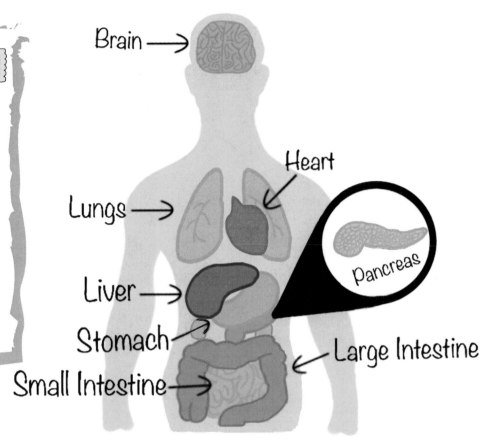

The pancreas is an organ that is behind your stomach. It has two purposes. One is that it helps breakdown food when it leaves the stomach. The other purpose is to create two hormones, insulin and glucagon. These hormones help control the amount of sugar in our blood.

A lot of things changed when Anna got diagnosed with type 1 diabetes, but a lot didn't.

She can still sing and dance.

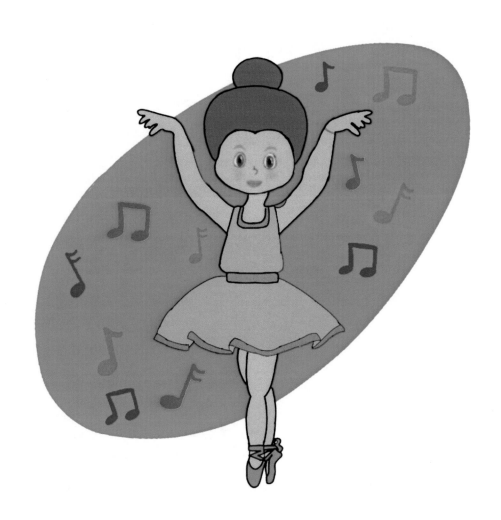

She can still laugh so hard
she cries.

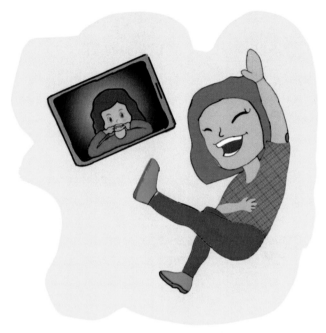

She can still run
and play.

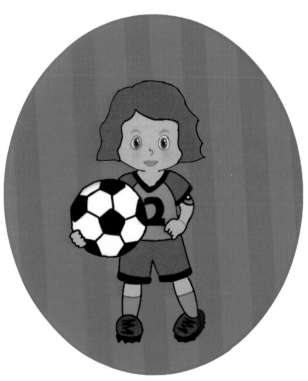

No matter how difficult diabetes seems,
it can not take away her hopes and dreams.

After Anna was diagnosed with type 1 diabetes, I discovered that there are over one million children and over eight million adults worldwide who have this disease. Even though there are so many people with this disorder, if there were 1000 people in a room, only one of them is likely to have type 1 diabetes.

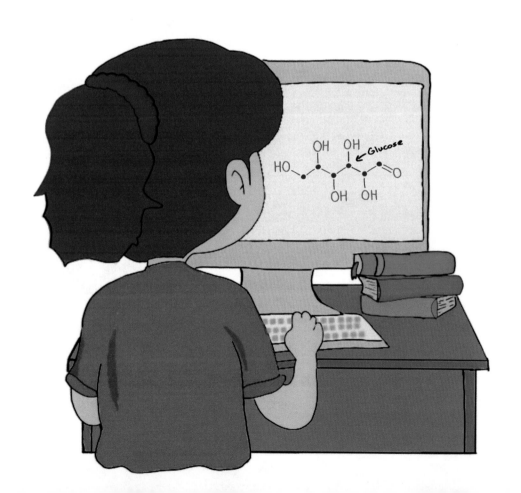

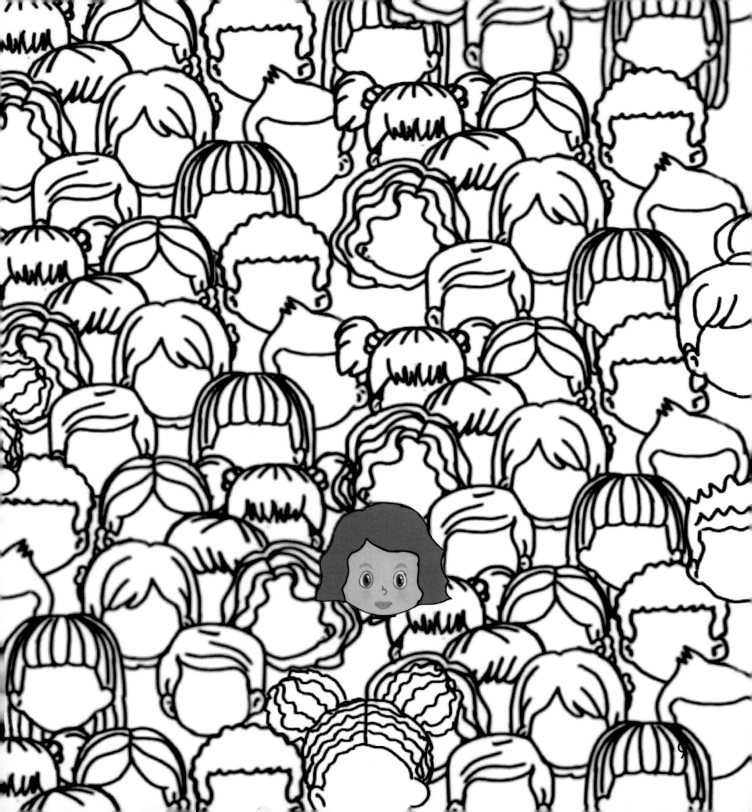

Type 1 diabetes is manageable but it does come with its challenges. When Anna was diagnosed with diabetes, it turned her world upside down. When something big changes, what you do every day changes too.

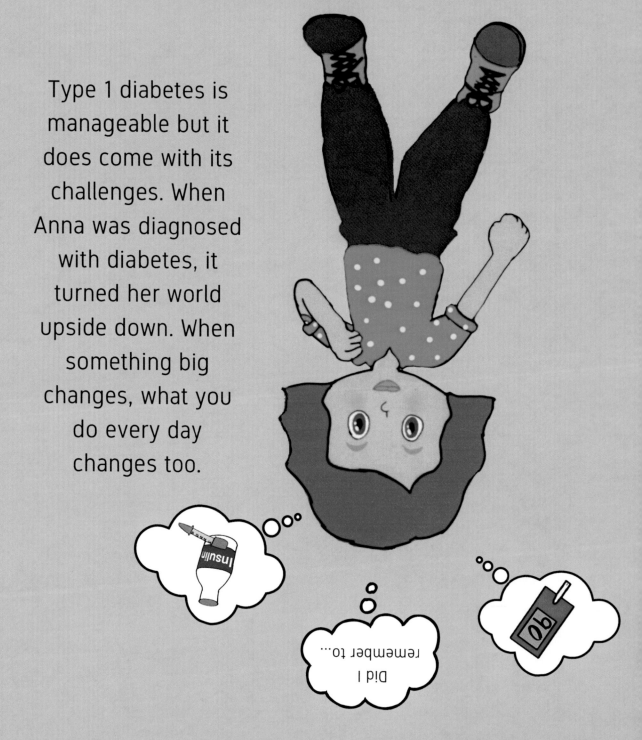

Anna needs to eat a well balanced diet that includes a variety of healthy foods. The sugar we eat is broken down into smaller parts. One of these parts is glucose. Anna must keep track of her glucose levels throughout the day. Watching what she eats and checking her glucose helps her decide how much insulin she needs to take. Taking the correct amount of insulin keeps her blood sugar at the right level and helps her avoid the unpleasant symptoms of low and high blood sugar levels. It also helps Anna prevent diabetes complications.

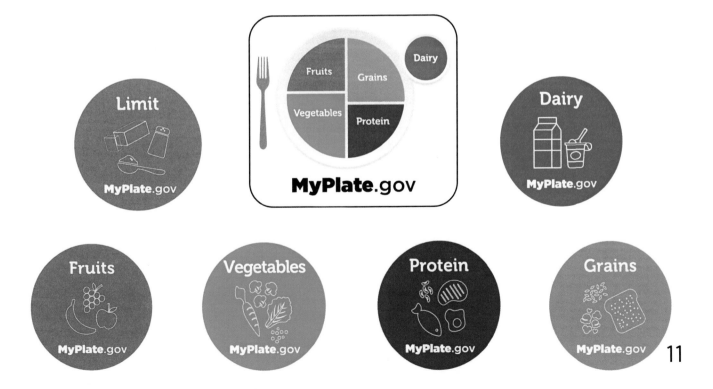

Anna has a continuous glucose monitor, which she wears on her arm. Every five minutes, it checks her glucose level. Anna uses this monitor by placing her phone in front of the sensor on her arm. Her phone then displays her current glucose level. Anna must replace the sensor on her arm every ten days. She uses a fancy patch to keep it in place. The patches come in a variety of colors and patterns. Anna's favorite patch is the pink camofulage one.

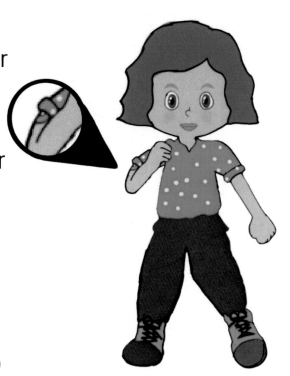

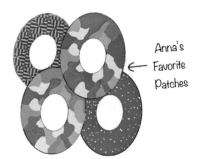

Anna's
← Favorite
Patches

Fun Fact

The first continuous glucose monitor was approved in 1999.

When Anna reads her glucose, it might be at the right level, but the monitor will warn her if it is likely to go up or down based on its previous readings. Knowing if her glucose is going to go low or high soon is very important to the management of Anna's type 1 diabetes.

Fun Fact

Service dogs have been trained to detect low blood sugar levels. These dogs use their sense of smell to detect low glucose levels and alert you when it is becoming low.

Anna also has a handheld glucose meter. She pricks her finger and places a small drop of blood on a test strip in the meter. The drop of blood and hole are so small that when Anna is done you would never know she had just pricked her finger. Anna has gotten use to the handheld meter and says it doesn't hurt but she prefers to use the glucose reader she has on her arm instead. Anna decides how much insulin she needs after reading her glucose level and reviewing how much food she has recently eaten.

Fun Fact

Animals can also get type 1 diabetes. Blood glucose levels in dogs and cats are similar to those in people. A range between 80 and 120 mg/dl is considered healthy.

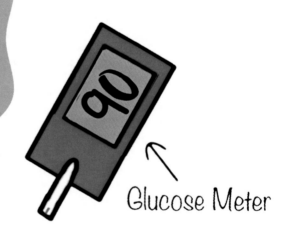

Glucose Meter

It is important that Anna knows how much sugar she eats. Sugar is in candy and dessert but there is also sugar in foods like bread, fruit, and pasta. Anna needs to keep track of all of the food she eats because this helps her know how much insulin she needs. Insulin is a medicine that diabetics use to help control their blood sugar level. This job is done automatically by the body for people who do not have diabetes, but because Anna's body does not produce insulin, she must decide how much insulin to take after each meal or snack.

Fun Fact

The insulin used to treat diabetes used to come from pigs and cows. Diabetics today use insulin that is made artificially.

My mom does not like to keep candy and sweets in the house because she says it is important for Anna and me to eat healthy. Anna and I have a massive sweet tooth. My mom will let us eat sweets once in a while and when she does, Anna needs to take extra insulin that day. If Anna has too many sweets and does not take enough insulin she gets hyperglycemia. This means her blood sugar is too high.

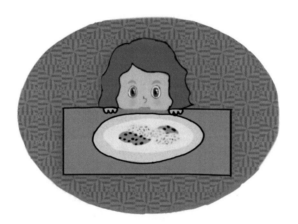

When Anna's blood sugar is high she usually feels drowsy and needs to pee more often. To get rid of these symptoms Anna needs to take more insulin but it can take hours or even a day for her to feel like her normal self again. Anna has to watch what she eats and monitor her glucose all of the time. If Anna has a big meal she takes more insulin and when she has a small meal she takes less insulin.

KNOW THE SIGNS OF
HYPERGLYCEMIA
HIGH BLOOD SUGAR

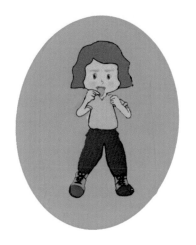

Dry Mouth

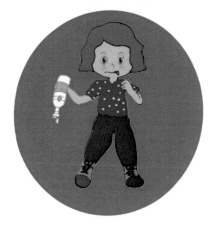

Extreme Thirst

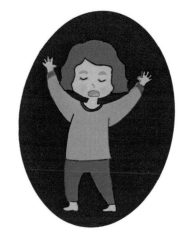

Drowsiness

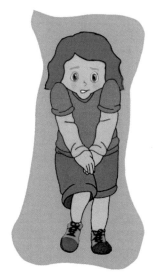

Frequent Urination

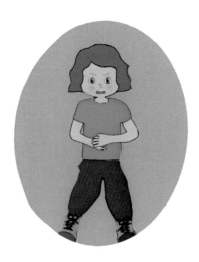

Stomach Pain

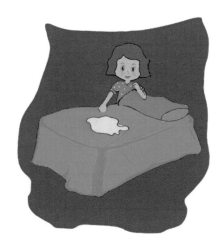

Bed Wetting

Anna uses an insulin pump to give herself insulin. It is a small electronic device that she wears. The device attaches to her skin. Anna usually places the insulin pump on her stomach but it can be attached in other places like her arm or leg. She can program the device to give specific amounts of insulin at different times of the day. She can also give herself extra insulin if she has a big meal or more sweets than usual.

Fun Fact

Some diabetics are beginning to use an artificial pancreas. This device monitors glucose levels in the body and automatically changes the amount of insulin delivered with little or no input from the patient.

Challenge Box

Is there a cure for type I diabetes?

HINT: People with type 1 diabetes need to take insulin for the rest of their lives.

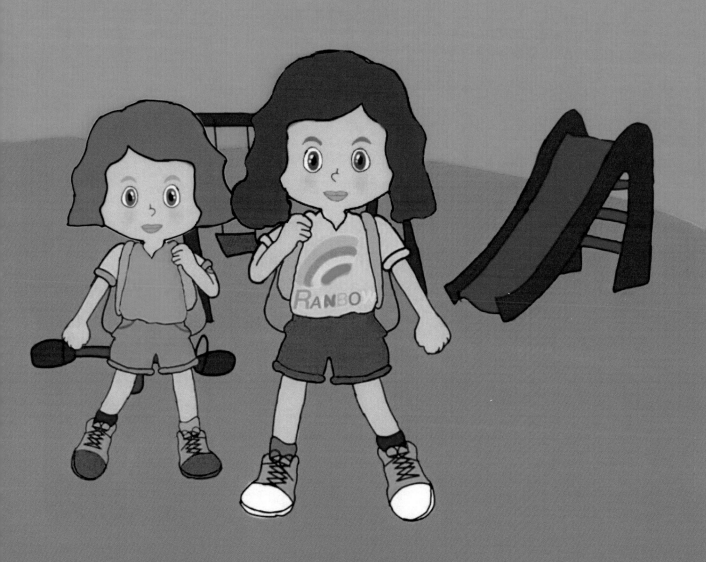

Anna tries to remember to check her glucose level before starting to play with her friends.

BEEP, BEEP, BEEP

If Anna takes too much insulin or forgets to eat, her glucose level may become dangerously low. When Anna's blood sugar drops, her phone beeps to alert her. When it goes off in school, she gets embarrassed, but everyone at school thinks she is cool, so they are glad she can take care of herself. When her phone beeps, all of her friends raise their hands hoping to be chosen by the teacher to walk her down to the nurse's office.

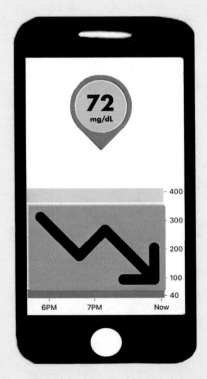

Fun Fact

Blood sugar levels change throughout the day. The changes are caused by how long ago you have eaten and what and how much you have eaten. Glucose levels can also be affected by activity level, stress, or illness.

Vocabulary

bat	mat	chat
cat	sat	that
rat	fat	gnat
hat	pat	flat

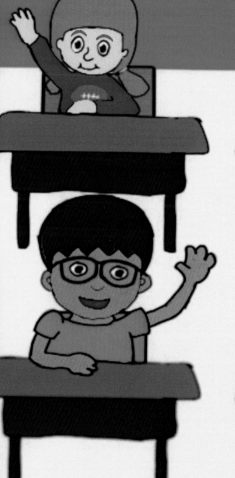

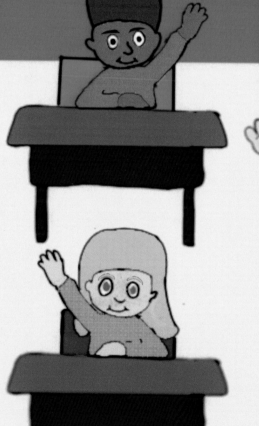

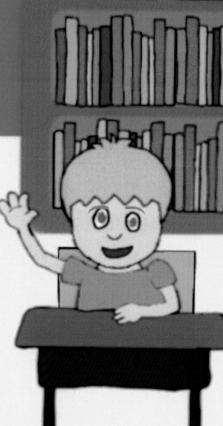

Anna forgot her phone at home one day so she was not alerted when her glucose level was getting low. A low glucose level is called hypoglycemia. Anna becomes tired and confused when she has hypoglycemia. Even though she has these symptoms Anna does not always recognize this may be happening to her. On the day Anna forgot her phone she did not realize her sugar was getting low. She was yawning and acting confused. She was with her friend Jackson drawing in art class. Jackson could tell Anna was having difficulty with her artwork. Thankfully, the students had learned about hypoglycemia symptoms. Jackson raised his hand and Mrs. Jones came over to where he and Anna were sitting. She noticed Anna sweating even though the classroom was chilly. Sweating is another symptom of hypoglycemia. Mrs. Jones decided Anna should visit the nurse's office.

KNOW THE SIGNS OF
HYPOGLYCEMIA
LOW BLOOD SUGAR

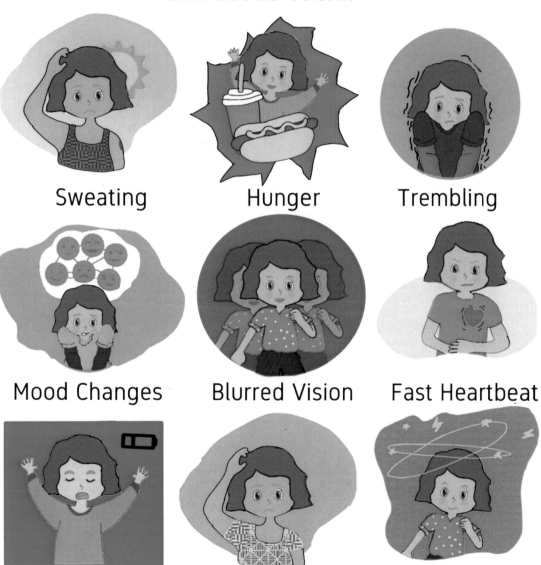

Sweating   Hunger   Trembling

Mood Changes   Blurred Vision   Fast Heartbeat

Tired and Pale   Headache   Dizziness or Confusion

23

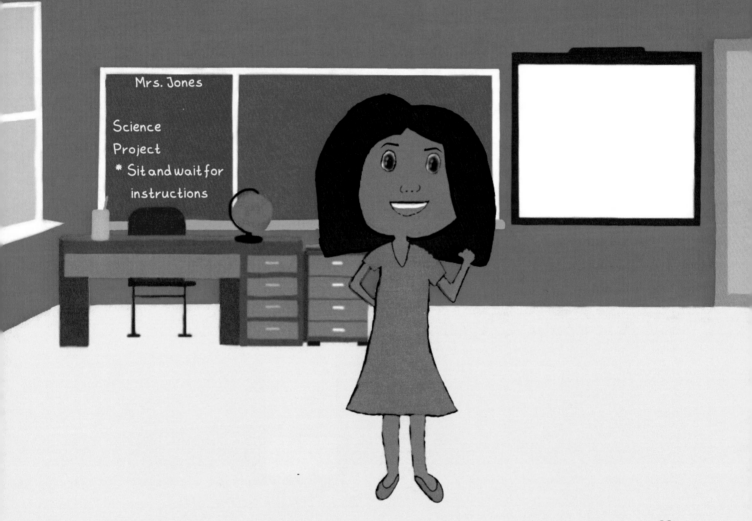

Mrs. Jones asked Jackson to bring Anna to the nurse's office.

24

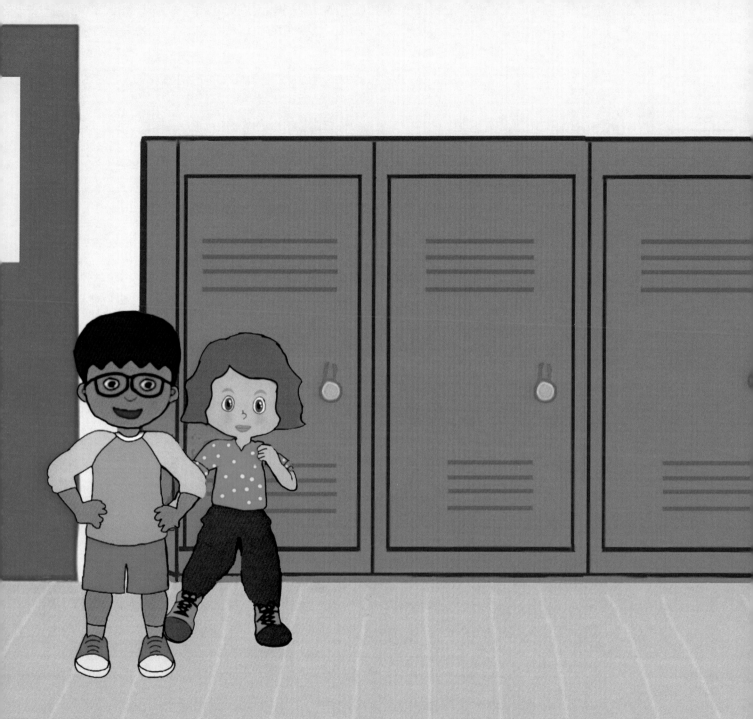

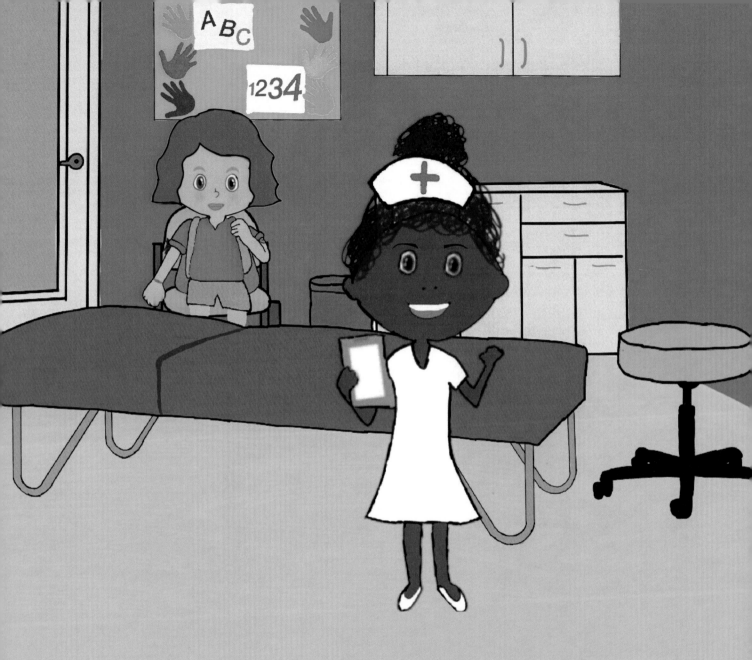

Nurse Patty uses Anna's handheld glucose meter
to check her glucose level.

Nurse Patty gives Anna a glucose tab that she keeps in her office. Glucose tabs look like old grandma candy and come in a variety of flavors. They help raise Anna's glucose level quickly. Anna enjoys visiting the nurse's office because there are always fun toys there. She can play with the toys while she waits for the glucose tab to work. She returns to class once her glucose level returns to normal and she feels well.

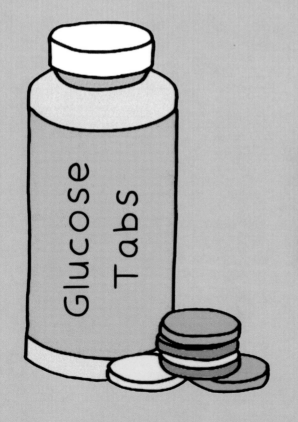

Fun Fact

If glucose tabs are not available, fruit juice, regular soda, milk, or sugary candy can be used to treat hypoglycemia.

Anna worries that if her glucose level drops, the people around her will not know what to do. I reassure her, that her medical alert bracelet will let other people know that she has type 1 diabetes. The silver medical alert bracelet has a small red plus on the outside. Anna's name is written on the inside of the bracelet. It also states that she is a type 1 diabetic and lists my parents' phone number, so they can be reached in an emergency.

Fun Fact

A medical alert bracelet can list your name, allergies, medications, and other details. First responders are trained to inspect their patient's wrist for a medical ID bracelet.

MEDICAL
+
ALERT

Challenge Box

Can you tell someone has type 1 diabetes by looking at them?

HINT: This is the reason medical alert bracelets are important.

Anna has learned to live with diabetes. She takes care of herself in order to live a long and healthy life. Anna hopes when she grows up she can be a scientist so that she can find a cure for this disease. She dreams of the day when no one will have to worry about type 1 diabetes.

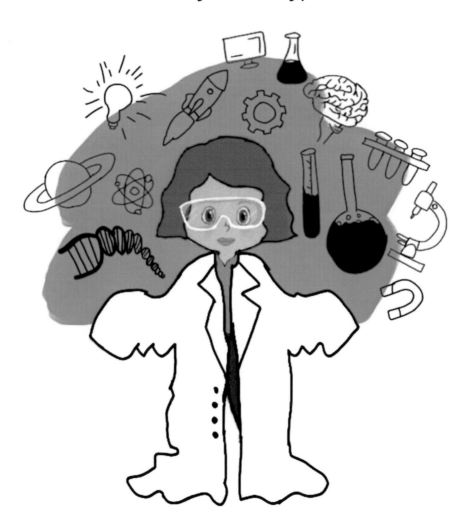

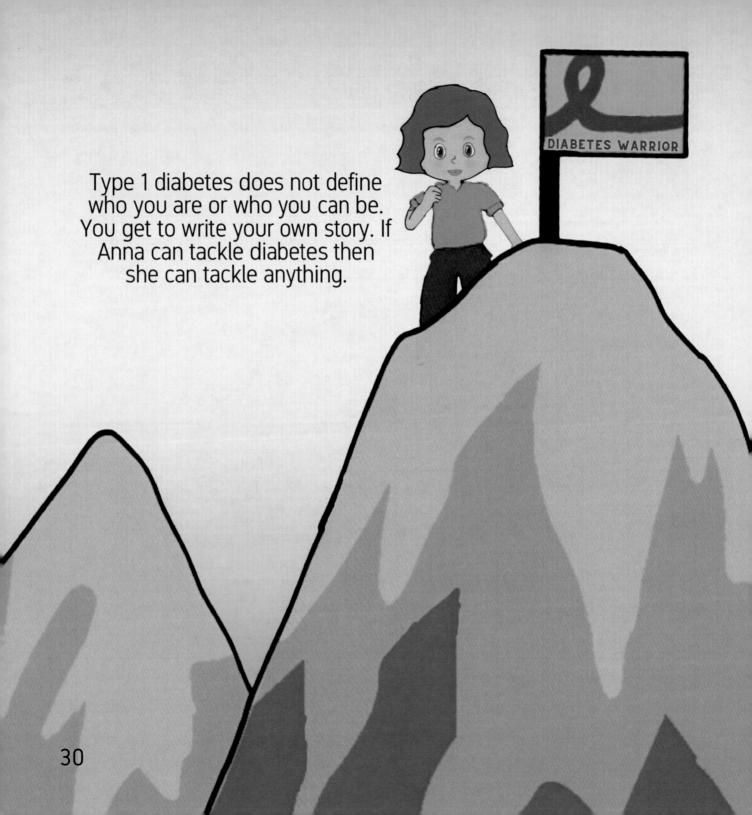

Type 1 diabetes does not define who you are or who you can be. You get to write your own story. If Anna can tackle diabetes then she can tackle anything.

Made in United States
North Haven, CT
17 April 2023